My Mediterranean Salads Collection

50 Ideas for Special Mediterranean Salads

Mateo Buscema

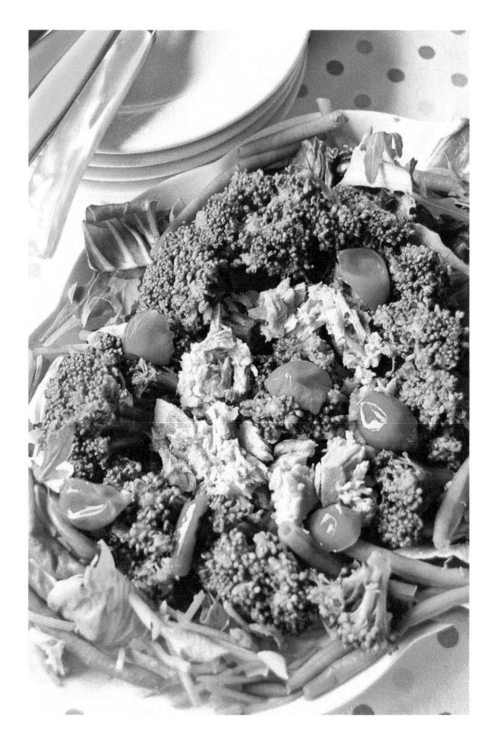

TABLE OF CONTENTS

Mediterranean power lentil salad

This recipe blends several vegetables mainly spinach and other crunchy veggies and pomegranate seeds for a perfect vegan meal.

Directions

- 2 teaspoon of honey
- Seeds of 1 pomegranate
- Salt and pepper
- Water
- 1 cup of chopped fresh parsley
- Kosher salt
- 1 teaspoon of ground cumin
- 1 small red onion chopped
- ¾ cucumber small diced
- ½ teaspoon of ground allspice
- 3 cups of baby spinach
- 1 cup of dry green lentils or black lentils
- Crumbled feta cheese for garnish
- ¼ cup of fresh lime juice
- ⅓ cup of extra virgin olive oil

Directions

1. In a medium sized saucepan, combine lentils with water (3 cups) and a pinch of kosher salt.

2. Bring to a boil.

3. Reduce heat to medium-low and allow it to simmer until the lentils are tender in 45 minutes.

4. Drain any excess water and set aside for later.

5. In a large separate mixing bowl, combine the cooked lentils together with the chopped onions, baby spinach, cucumbers, parsley, and pomegranate seeds and toss.

6. In another different small bowl, whisk together lime juice, extra virgin olive oil, honey, cumin, allspice, salt and pepper.

7. Pour this dressing over the lentil salad and toss.

8. Add a sprinkle of feta cheese to finish.

9. Give it some minutes to melt the flavors.

10. Serve and enjoy.

Mediterranean orange and pomegranate salad

This recipe is so refreshing with mint and honey dressing.

It features pomegranate seeds and slices of sweet oranges.

Ingredients

- 1 tablespoon of extra virgin olive oil
- 1 ½ ounces of thinly sliced red onions
- 25 fresh mint leaves, chopped
- 6 Navel oranges, peeled, sliced into rounds
- Pinch kosher salt
- 1 tablespoon of honey
- Pinch of sweet paprika
- pinch ground cinnamon
- Seeds of 1 pomegranate
- 1 lime, juice of lemon
- 1 ½ teaspoon of orange blossom water

Directions

1. In a small bowl, mix together the lime juice with the olive oil, honey and orange blossom water. Keep aside.

2. Place the sliced onions in a bowl of ice cold water.

3. Set aside for 10 minutes.

4. Remove the onions from the water and pat dry completely.

5. Sprinkle half of the amount of chopped mint leaves on the platter.

6. Arrange the orange slices and onions on top.

7. Sprinkle with a pinch of salt, sweet paprika, and cinnamon.

8. Next, spread the pomegranate seeds on top.

9. Drizzle the dressing over the orange pomegranate salad.

10. Top the salad with the remaining fresh mint leaves.

11. Keep aside for 5 minutes.

12. Serve and enjoy.

Fattoush salad

Salad is the king in all Mediterranean Sea diet dishes.

This is a simple salad recipe dressed in zesty lime vinaigrette served with pita chips.

Ingredients

- 2 cups of chopped fresh parsley leaves, stems removed
- 1½ teaspoon of sumac , more for later
- Salt and pepper
- 1 heart of Romaine lettuce, chopped
- scant ¼ teaspoon of ground allspice
- 1 English cucumber, chopped
- Early harvest extra virgin olive oil
- ¼ teaspoon of ground cinnamon
- 5 Roma tomatoes, chopped
- 2 loaves of pita bread
- 1 ½ lime, juice of lemon
- 5 green onions chopped
- 5 radishes, stems removed, thinly sliced
- 1 cup of chopped fresh mint leaves (optional)

Directions

1. Toast the pita bread in the toaster oven until it is crisp.
2. Heat 3 tablespoon of olive oil in a large pan.
3. Break the pita bread into pieces, and place in the heated oil.
4. Fry briefly until browned, tossing frequently.
5. Add salt, pepper and ½ teaspoon of sumac .
6. Remove the pita chips from the heat and drain on paper towels.
7. In a large mixing bowl, combine the chopped lettuce, tomatoes, cucumber, green onions with the sliced radish and parsley.
8. To make the dressing, whisk together the lemon or lime juice, olive oil and spices in a small bowl.
9. Dress the salad with the dressing and toss lightly.
10. Add the pita chips.
11. Transfer to small serving bowls.
12. Serve and enjoy.

Balela salad

This is a massive and wholesome salad packed with nutritious chickpeas and chopped vegetables and flavors from various herbs and lemon and garlic.

Ingredients

- ½ cup of freshly chopped parsley leaves
- ½ green bell pepper, cored and chopped
- Salt and black pepper
- 1 jalapeno, finely chopped
- ½ teaspoon of crushed red pepper
- 2 ½ cups grape tomatoes slice in halves
- 1 teaspoon of ground sumac
- 5 green onions, both white and green parts, chopped
- ½ cup of sun-dried tomatoes
- ½ teaspoon of Aleppo pepper
- ⅓ cup of pitted Kalamata olives
- 3 ½ cups of cooked chickpeas
- ¼ cup of pitted green olives
- ½ cup of freshly chopped mint or basil leaves
- ¼ cup of early harvest Greek extra virgin olive oil
- 2 tablespoons of white wine vinegar
- 2 tablespoons of lemon juice

- 1 garlic clove, minced

Directions

1. In a large bowl, mix together chickpeas, vegetables, sun-dried tomatoes, olives, and fresh herbs.
2. In a separate smaller bowl, mix together the extra virgin olive oil, white wine vinegar, lemon juice, minced garlic, salt and pepper, and spices.
3. Drizzle the dressing over the salad and mix to coat.
4. Leave aside for 30 minutes.
5. Cover and refrigerate until ready to serve.
6. Mix and taste to adjust the seasoning.
7. Serve and enjoy.

Stuffed grape leaves

The stuffed grape leaves are a fantastic tantalizing mixture of rice featuring fresh herbs and variety of vegetables mainly grape leaves.

This makes this recipe vegetarian and pure Mediterranean Sea diet.

Ingredients

- 1 ½ cup of short grain rice
- Extra virgin olive oil
- ½ teaspoon of cumin
- Juice of 2 lemons
- 2 tomatoes sliced into rounds
- About 4 cups of low-sodium chicken broth
- Kosher salt
- Black pepper
- 1 tsp allspice
- 12 ounces of lean ground beef
- 1 large yellow onion, finely chopped
- 1 16 ounces of jar grape leaves in brine
- ½ cup of chopped fresh parsley, fresh dill, and fresh mint

Directions

1. Firstly, soak the rice in plenty of water for 20 minutes. Drain.
2. As the rice cooks, heat 1 tablespoon of extra virgin olive oil in a large skillet.
3. Add onions and cook briefly, tossing until translucent.
4. Add the meat and cook till fully browned, toss.
5. Drain any excess fat, then season with kosher salt, pepper, and spices and toss.
6. Remove from heat and set aside to cool.
7. In a mixing bowl, combine the meat, drained rice, and fresh herbs.
8. Season lightly with kosher salt.
9. Drizzle with extra virgin olive oil, and mix.
10. Brush the bottom of a heavy pot with extra virgin olive oil.
11. Organize some grape leaves in the bottom. Top with sliced tomatoes.
12. Place one grape leave on a cutting board the textured side facing up.
13. Take 1 heaping teaspoon of the filling and place in the center of the leave, then fold the sides over the filling and roll. Repeat this step with remaining leaves.
14. Arrange the grape leaves in row, in your prepared pot, covering the circumference of the pot.
15. Then place a small plate inverted on top.

16. Boil the broth, pour over the grape leaves, arriving at the top layer and somewhat covering.

17. Cover and cook over medium heat for 30 minutes.

18. Add the juice of 2 lemons. Cover again with the lid, cook on low heat for 45 minutes.

19. Remove from heat. Allow to rest uncovered for 20 minutes.

20. Serve and enjoy with lemon wedges.

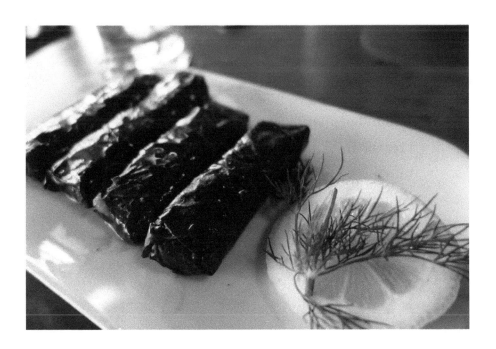

Simple Mediterranean cucumber salad

This is a simple yet loaded with freshness and bright for a salad.

It features shallots, dill and a lemon juice for a flavor.

Ingredients

- Juice of ½ lemon
- 2 shallots thinly sliced
- 6 radishes thinly sliced
- Salt and pepper
- 1 teaspoon of dried oregano
- ¼ ounces of chopped fresh dill
- 4 tablespoon of extra virgin olive oil
- 2 cucumbers thinly sliced
- 2 tablespoon of white wine vinegar

Directions

1. Place sliced cucumbers in a large mixing bowl.
2. Add sliced shallots, radish, and fresh dill.

3. In a small bowl, combine the extra virgin olive oil with white wine vinegar, lemon juice, oregano, kosher salt and black pepper.
4. Whisk until well combined.
5. Pour the dressing over the salad. Toss again.
6. Serve and enjoy.

Fresh Mediterranean bean salad

Beans are an ingredient fully packed with protein nutrients.

It is greatly flavored with herbs, capers and garlic.

Ingredients

- 2 garlic cloves minced
- 1 15- oz. can garbanzo beans chickpeas, drained and rinsed
- ½ tablespoon of Dijon mustard
- 1 green bell pepper cored and chopped
- 1 red bell pepper cored and chopped
- ½ cucumber diced
- Salt and black pepper
- 1 cup of chopped red onions
- 1 ½ tablespoons of capers
- 1 15 oz. can kidney beans drained and rinsed
- 1 cup of chopped fresh parsley
- 15 fresh mint leaves torn
- 2 tablespoons of lemon juice
- 1 15- oz. can cannellini beans drained and rinsed
- 15 fresh basil leaves torn
- 1 teaspoon of sugar
- ¼ cup of extra virgin olive oil

Directions

1. In a large mixing bowl, combine the beans together with the chopped peppers, onions, capers and fresh herbs. Mix.

2. In another small separate bowl, add the garlic, Dijon mustard, lemon juice, sugar, extra virgin olive oil, and salt and pepper. Whisk combine.

3. Add the vinaigrette to the salad bowl. Toss to coat.

4. Cover and refrigerate for a bit to soak the vinaigrette into the beans.

5. Serve and enjoy.

Quick pickled cucumber recipe

This recipe again blends the flavors of garlic and dill including green onions with jalapeno making it a perfect salad.

Ingredients

- 2 ½ tablespoons of kosher salt
- 6 garlic cloves minced
- 3 tablespoon of peppercorn
- 2 bay leaves
- Few sprigs of fresh dill
- 3 tablespoon of mustard seed
- 3 cups of vinegar distilled white vinegar
- 1 ¼ lb. of Persian cucumbers
- 2 ¼ cup of cold water
- 3 tablespoon of coriander seed
- 4 green onions trimmed and chopped
- 3 Jalapeno peppers sliced into rounds

Directions

1. In a saucepan, combine the vinegar together with water, coriander seed, mustard seed, peppercorn, salt, and bay leaves.

2.   Boil over high heat.

3.   Reduce the heat, let simmer for 10 minutes. let cool.

4.   Pack the cucumbers together with the green onions, jalapenos, garlic, and a few springs of dill in some wide jars.

5.   Ladle the brine into the jars to cover the cucumbers.

6.   Give the jars a couple of taps to release any air bubbles and allow the cubes to settle.

7.   Cover the jars tightly with their lids and refrigerate.

8.   Serve and enjoy.

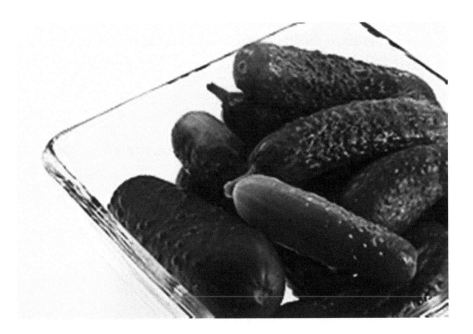

Vegan stuffing

This recipe is 100% vegetarian perfect for a Mediterranean diet easily customizable with extras.

Ingredients can be substituted with one's favorites.

It only takes approximately 55 minutes to get ready.

Ingredients

- 8 cups of diced bread, dried overnight
- 2 tablespoons of olive oil
- 2 teaspoons of dried thyme
- 1 small onion, minced
- 2.5 cups of button mushrooms, quartered
- 1 cup of pomegranate seeds
- 2 celery stalks, diced
- 1 green apple, diced
- 1 teaspoon of dried rosemary , finely chopped
- 2 cups of vegetable broth

Directions

1. Start by preheating your oven to 350°F.
2. As your oven is heating, add and heat oil in a frying pan.

3. Add minced onion together with the quartered mushrooms, diced celery, let sauté for 10 minutes as you stir occasionally.
4. Add rosemary, thyme and mix well.
5. Move the mixture to a large mixing dis.
6. Add dried bread together with the apple.
7. Pour over 1 cup of broth. Mix to combine.
8. Shift it to a baking dish and add more broth if desired.
9. In the preheated oven, cook for 40 minutes, stir infrequently.
10. Serve and enjoy.

Watermelon feta salad with cherries

Watermelon is a perfect choice for this fruity recipe and for a Mediterranean Sea diet.

It is best for BBQ parties or even picnics or any outdoor event.

Ingredients

- 2 ears of corn on the cob
- 10 ounces of fresh cherries
- 4 pounds of watermelon
- 3 tablespoon of butter
- Salt to taste
- ½ lemon, juice only
- Fresh mint, see note 4
- 3.5 ounces of feta cheese

Directions

1. In a boiling water, cook corn without silk threads for 10 minutes.
2. Transfer to a plate when ready to let cool.

3. As the corn cooks, pit and cut the cherries and watermelon into chunks respectively.
4. Place in a serving dish.
5. Cut off kernels and shift the content to a pan with butter, roast for 5 minutes.
6. Season with salt.
7. Then drizzle with lemon juice.
8. The roasted kernels should then be poured over the watermelon and cherries.
9. Serve and enjoy when topped with crumbled feta cheese and mint leaves.

Buckwheat salad

This recipe is good for breakfast or easy quick lunch.

It a Mediterranean gluten free recipe that would be loved by any vegetarian or vegan.

Ingredients

- 1.5 cup of cherry tomatoes
- ¾ cup of buckwheat, uncooked
- 1.5 cup of water
- a generous pinch of black pepper
- 1 tablespoon of extra virgin olive oil
- 1 teaspoon of salt
- 4 – 5 sprigs fresh flat leaf parsley
- ½ cucumber
- 1 large yellow pepper

Directions

1. Place the buckwheat in a small sauce pan.
2. Add the water and salt to it and boil.
3. Lower the heat to low let simmer for a 15 minutes.
4. Drain any excess water.
5. Cut vegetables into small chunks.

6. Shift them into a mixing bowl

7. Season with salt and pepper.

8. Add olive oil on it then sprinkle with finely chopped parsley mix well.

9. Taste and season accordingly.

10. Serve and best enjoy warm.

Apple chickpeas salad

This celery, apples and pan-roasted chickpea are the main ingredients of this Mediterranean Sea diet recipe.

It is dressed with avocado and peanut butter.

Ingredients

- 14 ounce of cooked chickpea
- 1 tablespoon of soy sauce
- 2 tablespoons of peanut butter
- ½ cup of water
- ½ medium lemon, juice only
- a handful of fresh flat leaf parsley
- 1 tablespoon of paprika
- 4 medium apples
- 1 tablespoon of extra virgin olive oil
- 1 small ripe avocado
- 2 tablespoon of extra virgin olive oil
- 2 celery stalks
- ½ medium lemon, juice only

Directions

1. In a frying pan, heat oil until shimmering without smoke.

2. Add the chickpeas let roast for 4 minutes. Keep tossing.

3. Add paprika and the toasted chickpea toss to coat. Continue to roast briefly then turn off the heat.

4. Combine it with lemon juice and parsley.

5. Season it with a bit of salt and a pinch of pepper.

6. Cut and place the apples into a serving bowl with the roasted chickpea. Mix.

7. Put all the ingredients in a food processor or blend.

8. Process until when smooth.

9. Adjust thickness accordingly with water.

10. Serve and enjoy.

Goat cheese salad with walnut dressing

Ingredients

- 4 tablespoon of honey
- 12 ounces of iceberg lettuce
- 1 cup of croutons
- 6 ounces of tomatoes
- 6 tablespoon of extra virgin olive oil
- 6 ounces of cucumber
- ¼ cup of water
- Goat cheese to your taste
- 3.5 ounces of walnuts

Directions

1. Clean the vegetables and cut into pieces.
2. Place all of them in a mixing bowl.
3. Process the walnut in a food processor.
4. Add olive oil together with the honey and water. Mix to combine.
5. Serve and enjoy.

Fresh fruit salad with coconut honey dressing

This recipe involves the combination of variety of fruits according to one's choice and flavoring them with syrup.

Ingredients

- 1 cup white grapes
- 1 cup blackberries
- 5 tablespoons honey
- 2 cups watermelon, cubes
- 1 medium lemon
- 5 tablespoons coconut oil
- ½ sugar melon
- ½ cantaloupe melon

Directions

1. Clean and cut the watermelon flesh into cubes.
2. Place in the serving dish.
3. Cut the grapes in halves.
4. Place the grapes in a bowl with the blackberries.
5. Refrigerate until time for serving.

6. As it refrigerates, combine all the ingredients in a bowl.

7. Pour them over the salad.

8. Serve and enjoy chilled.

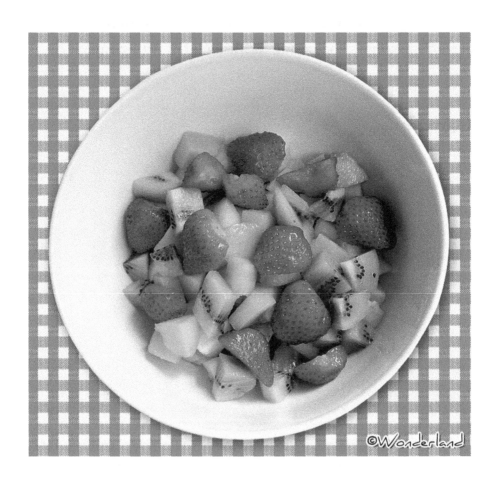

Shaved zucchini salad with walnuts

This recipe features seeds and a flavorful drizzle with lemon juice for a perfect easy side fresh vegetables.

Ingredients

- 1 tablespoon of black sesame seeds
- 1 small onion
- ¼ cup of mixed seeds
- 1 zucchini
- ¼ cup of walnuts , chopped
- Pinch of salt
- Carrot
- Fresh basil leaves
- 2 medium tomatoes
- ½ lemon

Directions

1. Prepare the vegetables and fruits by washing and peeling
2. Cut tomatoes and slice carrots.
3. Cut onions into rings.

4. Arrange all the ingredients on a plate.

5. Squeeze lemon juice over the salad

6. Season with salt and sprinkle with sesame seeds.

7. Use the basil leaves for garnishing.

8. Serve and enjoy.

Mediterranean green salad

This recipe is a perfect outdoor or entertainment recipe or grill parties.

It only takes 10 minutes.

Ingredients

- 1 butter lettuce
- 2 tablespoons of honey
- A few fresh mint leaves
- 1 tablespoon of lemon juice
- 2 spring onions
- 2 cups of fresh sweet peas
- 2 green peppers
- 1½ cup cherry tomatoes
- 5 tablespoons of extra virgin olive oil
- 1 cup of mange tout

Directions

1. Cut lettuce into thin strips
2. Shell the peas.
3. Slice the spring onions.
4. Cut green peppers into thin strips.

5. Half the tomatoes.

6. Combine all the ingredients i.e. olive oil, chopped mint leaves. lemon juice, and honey.

7. Pour over the salad.

8. Serve and enjoy.

Strawberry salad with poppy seeds dressing

This recipe is a typical side dish for a BBQ combined with strawberries, spring onions and lettuce.

It gets ready in only 10 minutes.

Ingredients

- 1 tablespoon of balsamic reduction
- 4 tablespoons of extra virgin olive oil
- 2 cups of fresh strawberries
- 2 tablespoons of poppy seeds
- 1 head of butter lettuce
- 2 spring onions

Directions

1. Clean and chop the ingredients and place them in a serving dish.
2. Mix them together with hands.
3. Combine extra virgin olive oil, poppy seeds, and balsamic reduction. Mix well in a jar.
4. Pour the mixture over the salad.

5. Serve and enjoy immediately.

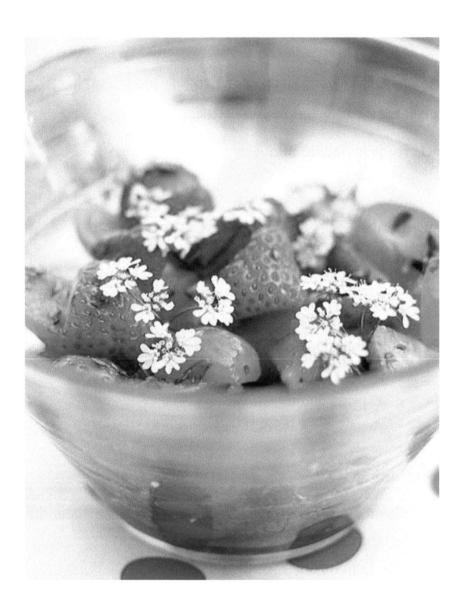

Chick salad with lima beans, beets and spinach

This recipe is crunchy, sweet with a vibrant color packed with fiber, mineral, and vitamins.

It also serves as a great appetizer for a dull meal.

Ingredients

- 2 tablespoons of unsalted butter
- 5 radishes
- 2 chicken breasts
- 2 beets
- Salt and pepper
- 1 cup of fresh lima beans
- 1 can of sweetcorn
- 4 cups of fresh spinach

Directions

1. Place in a large pot and fill with water.
2. Bring to the boil.
3. Lower the heat after 40 minutes of boiling and let simmer for another 10 minutes.

4. Drain any excess water and allow it to cool.

5. Shell the pods.

6. Slice the radishes, put in a bowl together with spinach.

7. Next, slice your chicken breast into thin strips.

8. Season with salt.

9. Melt butter in a frying pan.

10. Place the chicken strips in the pan, let fry until golden brown.

11. Add the lima beans together with the sweetcorn.

12. Sauté for 3 minutes.

13. Season with black pepper.

14. Serve and enjoy.

Creamy potato and ham salad

Ingredients

- 1 lb. potatoes
- Black pepper
- 2 carrots, medium
- 5 ounces of dill pickles
- 4 medium eggs
- 2 teaspoons of salt
- ½ cup of mayonnaise
- 1 onion, medium
- 5 ounces of canned peas
- ¼ cup of sour cream
- 5 ounces of ham

Directions

1. Clean and peel the potatoes and carrots.
2. Place them in a pot.
3. Add the eggs and pour in water.
4. Add 2 teaspoons of salt, cover.
5. Let the water boil. Lower the heat to let simmer for 10 minutes.
6. Transfer the eggs into a bowl. Let cool in cold water.
7. Let the potatoes and carrots continue to cook until done.

8. Drain out any excess water, then chop the vegetables.

9. Chop the onion, drain the peas.

10. Drain and slice the dill pickles into small pieces and dice the ham.

11. Peel the eggs, cut into small pieces.

12. Move every content to a large dish. Mix properly.

13. Add the potatoes with bit of salt and black pepper.

14. Combine the mayonnaise with sour cream.

15. Stir into the salad until well combined.

16. Taste and adjust accordingly.

17. Refrigerate for many hours preferably overnight.

18. Serve and enjoy.

Chicken and cucumber salad with parsley

This recipe is like a powerhouse of protein mainly the chicken and chickpeas along with edamame.

It gets ready only in 15 minutes making 6 servings

Ingredients

- 4 cups of loosely packed arugula
- 1 teaspoon of kosher salt
- 1 cup of fresh baby spinach
- 2 tablespoons of fresh lemon juice
- 1 tablespoon of grated Parmesan cheese
- 1 cup of chopped cucumber
- ¼ teaspoon of black pepper
- ½ cup of extra virgin olive oil
- 1 medium garlic clove, smashed
- 2 cups of packed fresh flat-leaf parsley leaves
- 4 cups of shredded rotisserie chicken
- 1 tablespoon of toasted pine nuts
- 2 cups of cooked shelled edamame
- 1 can of unsalted chickpeas, drained and rinsed

Directions

1. Combine together parsley with spinach, cheese, pine nuts, garlic, lemon juice, salt, and pepper in the dish of a food processor.
2. Blend or process until very smooth in 1 – 2 minutes.
3. As the processor is still operating, add oil blend for 1 more minute.
4. Stir chicken together with the chickpeas, edamame, and cucumber in a bowl or dish.
5. Add pesto, toss.
6. Put arugula in every bowl topping with the mixture of chicken.
7. Serve and enjoy immediately.

Shrimp, arugula, white beans, cherry tomato salad

This recipe is made up of a massive combination of healthy and tasty vegetables making it a perfect tasty Mediterranean Sea recipe for a vegan.

Ingredients

- ¼ teaspoon of black pepper
- 1 cup of cherry tomatoes, halved or quartered
- ½ cup of finely diced red onion
- ¾ teaspoon of grated lemon zest
- 3 handfuls of baby arugula leaves
- 3 tablespoons of red wine vinegar
- 2 15-ounce cans of cannellini white beans, rinsed and drained
- 1 pound of 16-20 count shelled and deveined shrimp
- 2 cloves of minced garlic
- ½ teaspoon of salt
- 3 tablespoons of extra virgin olive oil

Directions

1. Heat a large skillet over high heat.
2. Add 2 teaspoons of olive oil to coat pan.
3. In batches, add the shrimp, sauté for 1 minute on every side to sear when the oil is hot enough.
4. Remove from pan when almost ready, keep to cool.
5. Place drained beans, lemon zest, diced onion, cherry tomatoes, and arugula leaves into a large bowl.
6. Fold in the shrimp.
7. In another separate small bowl, whisk red wine vinegar together with the olive oil, garlic, salt, and pepper.
8. Make a fold of the dressing into the salad.
9. Serve and enjoy.

Vegan chopped chickpea Greek salad

Unlike other recipes, this vegan chopped chickpea Greek salad and other veggie salads does not need cooking at all.

As a result, everything is prepared and consumed raw for a typical Mediterranean Sea vegan diet.

Ingredients

- 1 medium bell pepper thinly sliced
- 1 medium red onion thinly sliced
- 2 cups of cherry tomatoes halved
- 1 cup of black olives sliced
- 1 large avocado
- ¼ teaspoon of salt
- ¼ cup of olive oil
- ½ teaspoon of Italian seasoning
- 8 cups of baby spinach
- 3 teaspoon of balsamic vinegar
- 1 teaspoon of lemon juice
- 1 can of chickpeas drained and rinsed
- 1 teaspoon of honey or date syrup
- 1 large cucumber sliced

- 1 teaspoon of Dijon mustard

Directions

1. First, add olive oil, vinegar, lemon juice, honey, Dijon mustard, and salt in a jar.
2. Shake well to combine.
3. Arrange all veggies and chickpeas on beds of spinach.
4. Add avocado and dressing right.
5. Serve and enjoy.

Mediterranean pasta salad

This pasta salad is a perfect meal for light lunch or dinner although it takes up to 4 hours to get ready.

In a nutshell, patience is highly recommended.

Ingredients

- 1 teaspoon of kosher salt
- 1 ½ cup of crumbled feta cheese
- 1 pint of grape tomatoes, sliced in half
- ½ teaspoon of ground black pepper
- 1 cup of Kalamata olives, pitted, coarsely chopped
- 1 cup of green olives, pitted, coarsely chopped
- ½ red onion, diced
- 1 large cucumber, diced
- 5 ounces of hard salami, sliced
- 1 pound of dried fusilli
- 1/3 cup of olive oil
- 1/8 cup of balsamic vinegar
- 1 tablespoon of granulated sugar
- 2 cloves of garlic, finely minced

Directions

1. Start by cooking pasta as directed on the package.

2. Drain excess water and put in a large bowl.

3. Add tomatoes, cucumber, olives, feta, red onion, and top with salami.

4. In another separate small bowl, whisk olive oil with garlic, sugar, balsamic vinegar, salt, and pepper.

5. Pour over pasta mixture, toss to coat.

6. Refrigerate for 4 hours or more.

7. Serve and enjoy when the time is up.

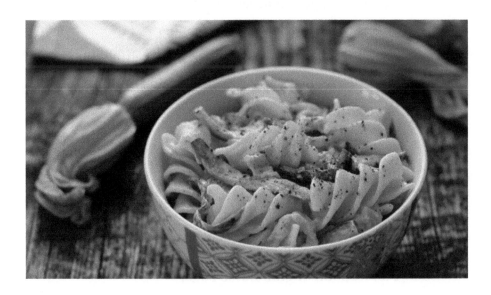

Horiatiki salata

Ingredients

- 1 large cucumber, peeled and sliced
- ½ teaspoon of oregano
- Splash of red wine vinegar
- ¼ red onion, cut into thin strips
- Salt and pepper
- 10 Kalamata olives
- 3 medium tomatoes, quartered
- 6 ounces of feta cheese
- ¼ cup of extra virgin olive oil
- ¼ red bell pepper, cut into thin strips

Directions

1. Add all veggies together with the olives to a bowl.
2. Top with olive oil, feta cheese, vinegar, and oregano.
3. Add salt and pepper
4. Serve and enjoy.

Greek kale salad with creamy tahini dressing

This Mediterranean Sea diet recipe features very bold Mediterranean flavors making it a healthier and tastier recipe.

Ingredients

- Freshly ground black pepper
- ½ cup of thinly sliced Kalamata olives
- ⅓ cup of finely grated Parmesan
- ⅓ cup of sunflower seeds
- ¼ teaspoon of extra-virgin olive oil
- 3 tablespoons of lemon juice
- 1 tablespoon of extra-virgin olive oil
- 1 medium clove garlic, pressed
- Fine sea salt
- ¼ cup of tahini
- ½ teaspoon of Dijon mustard
- ⅓ cup of oil-packed sun-dried tomatoes, rinsed and drained
- ¼ teaspoon of fine sea salt
- 1 can of chickpeas, rinsed and drained
- 2 tablespoons of water

- 1 medium bunch of curly green kale

Directions

1. Put chopped kale in a large serving bowl.
2. Sprinkle it lightly with salt and massage with your hands.
3. Add the chickpeas together with the olives and pepper rings, sun-dried tomatoes, and Parmesan keep aside.
4. Combine the sunflower seeds with the olive oil and a few dashes of salt in a small skillet over medium heat.
5. Let cook for 5 minutes, stirring frequently, until the seeds are turning lightly golden at the edges.
6. Pour the toasted seeds into the salad bowl.
7. In a small bowl, combine the tahini together with the olive oil, lemon juice, garlic, mustard, and salt.
8. Whisk to blend completely.
9. Add the water and whisk until blended.
10. Season with freshly black pepper.
11. Pour the dressing into the salad toss to equally coat the salad.
12. Serve and enjoy immediately.
13. Any leftovers can be refrigerated.

Vegetarian stuffed cabbage rolls

This cabbage is rolled with vegetarian rice filling loaded with various herbs and vegetables especially onions, tomatoes and spices to give the recipe a delicious taste.

Ingredients

- ¼ cup of extra virgin olive oil
- ½ cup of shredded yellow onion
- 2 Roma tomato sliced
- 1 tomato, chopped or diced
- 1 medium green cabbage
- 1 medium yellow onion sliced
- ½ cup of chopped fresh parsley
- ½ cup of chopped fresh dill
- 1 teaspoon of ground cumin
- Water
- ½ teaspoon of cayenne pepper
- ½ teaspoon of ground allspice
- Salt and pepper
- 1 15-oz. can of tomato sauce, divided
- 1 cup of long-grain rice

Directions

1. Remove and discard the first couple leaves of cabbage and clean in cold water.

2. Cut off the bottom then place the whole head of cabbage in boiling water, let boil 2 minutes.

3. Peel off the softened leaves, continue with the same process, peeling off the blanched layers of cabbage leaves as they soften.

4. Cut each cabbage leaf into halves, removing any thick veins.

5. In a large mixing bowl, combine the rice together with the shredded onions, herbs, spices, salt and pepper, chopped tomato, tomato sauce and water. Mix together.

6. Lightly oil a large heavy cooking pot.

7. Line the bottom with the sliced onions and sliced tomatoes.

8. Take a piece of cabbage and place on a flat surface, coarse side up.

9. Add 1 teaspoon of rice stuffing mixture at the end of the leaf closest to you.

10. Roll up the leaf to completely enclose the stuffing.

11. Repeat with all the remaining cabbage.

12. Layer the cabbage rolls, in the prepared pot.

13. Top with the remaining tomato sauce, and water.

14. Add a pinch of ground cumin.

15. Top the cabbage rolls with a small plate.

16. For 7 minutes, cook on high heat until the liquid reduces to half.
17. Lower the leaving the small plate in, and cover the pot with its own lid.
18. Continue to cook for 30 minutes, then remove the plate leave the lid to cover it.
19. Cook for more 15 minutes to absorb all the liquid.
20. Le the cabbage rolls rest for some time.
21. Serve and enjoy.

Herbed couscous recipe with roasted cauliflower

Herbs are another heart of the Mediterranean Sea diet.

As a result, this herbed couscous recipe with roasted cauliflower blends herbs with other flavors to give it a required taste to satisfy your taste buds.

Ingredients

For roasted cauliflower

- ½ teaspoon of black pepper
- Greek extra virgin olive oil
- 1 ½ teaspoon of sweet Spanish paprika
- ¾ teaspoon of cumin
- ¾ teaspoon of salt, more for later
- 1 head cauliflower, divided into small florets
- 1 ½ teaspoon of za'atar , more for later
- ½ teaspoon of cayenne pepper, optional

For Couscous

- 8 oz. uncooked pearl
- 1 3-Ingredient Mediterranean Salad
- 1 cup packed chopped fresh parsley

- Feta cheese
- 2 green onions, trimmed, both white and greens chopped
- Greek extra virgin olive oil
- 1 tahini sauce recipe
- 2 teaspoons of fresh lemon juice

Directions

1. Preheat oven to 475°F.
2. In a small bowl, spices, salt, and pepper.
3. Make sure to set aside 1 tablespoon of the spice mixture for later.
4. Place the cauliflower on a large sheet pan.
5. Drizzle with extra virgin olive oil.
6. Sprinkle the spice mixture on top of the cauliflower. Toss by hand to co\t well.
7. Spread on the sheet pan in one layer.
8. Cover the sheet pan with foil.
9. Place on the bottom rack of the heated oven.
10. Let bake for 10 minutes.
11. Remove from oven and uncover.
12. Return to heated oven, let bake for more 15 minutes.
13. Remove again from oven, turn cauliflower over on the other side.
14. Return to oven for another 12 minutes.

15. Prepare the simple Mediterranean salad normally. Prepare he tahini sauce normally.

16. In a saucepan, heat 1 tablespoon of extra virgin olive oil over medium heat.

17. Add couscous and the remaining 1 tablespoon of spice mixture.

18. Sauté, tossing regularly, until couscous is toasted into a light brown color.

19. Add boiling water. Turn heat to low, cover and simmer for 12 minutes or until liquid is absorbed and couscous is fully cooked.

20. Remove cooked couscous from heat source.

21. Add chopped green onions, parsley, and lemon juice. Mix.

22. Divide herbed couscous and roasted cauliflower among 4 dinner bowls.

23. Add 3-ingredient Mediterranean salad to each.

24. Sprinkle with feta cheese and a pinch of Za'atar.

25. Drizzle a little tahini over the cauliflower.

26. Serve and enjoy.

Fresh fava bean salad and fava spread

The flavor of this fresh fava bean is amazing with olive, lemon juice which can be turned to a delicious fava spread.

Ingredients

- 1 cup of bread cubes
- ½ cup of Kalamata olives, sliced
- ½ cup of chopped parsley
- 1 tablespoon of lemon juice, or to taste
- 2 tablespoons of olive oil
- 2 pounds of whole fresh fava beans in their pods
- 1 teaspoon of dried oregano
- Freshly ground black pepper to taste
- 3 tablespoons of olive oil

Directions

1. Start by preheat your oven ready to 350°F.
2. Then, brush the bread cubes with the olive oil.
3. Let bake for about 15 minutes or until the color turns golden.

4. Allow them to cool for 10 minutes.

5. Snap the fava pods in the meantime, and collect the fava beans in a bowl.

6. Set a medium pot filled with water over high heat.

7. Bring to a boil.

8. Then, add the fava beans let boil for 1 minute.

9. Drain any excess water with a colander, make sure to rinse with cold water until fava beans are no longer warm.

10. Now, cut the top of the membrane of each bean with a paring knife.

11. Squeeze it all with your fingers.

12. Make sure the bean can easily slide out quickly and swiftly.

13. Repeat this with all of the remaining beans.

14. Mix the shelled fava beans together with the croutons and the rest of the ingredients in a bowl.

15. After mixing, serve in your eating dish and enjoy immediately or when still warm.

Mega crunchy romaine salad with quinoa

Ingredient

For the Salad

- 1 ⅓ cups of water
- ½ teaspoon of olive oil
- ½ cup of chopped radishes
- ⅔ cup of uncooked quinoa, rinsed
- 1 small head of romaine
- ½ cup of raw sunflower seeds
- 1 cup of shredded carrots
- 1 cup of chopped cabbage
- ½ cup of dried cranberries

For the Zippy cilantro dressing

- ¼ cup of lightly packed fresh cilantro
- 2 teaspoons of honey or maple syrup
- ¼ teaspoon of chipotle chili powder
- 2 medium cloves garlic, roughly chopped
- ⅓ cup of olive oil
- ½ teaspoon of fine-grain sea salt
- 2 tablespoons of rice vinegar
- 3 tablespoons of lime juice

Directions

1. Combine the quinoa together with the water in a medium saucepan.
2. Bring to a boil over medium-high heat.
3. Lower the heat a bit to maintain a gentle simmer.
4. Let cook until the quinoa has absorbed all of the liquid in 15 minutes.
5. Reduce the heat further as time goes on to maintain a gentle simmer.
6. Remove the pot from heat.
7. Then, cover let the steam for 5 minutes, set aside for later.
8. Combine the sunflower seeds and olive oil in a medium skillet.
9. Let cook over medium heat, keep stirring frequently till the seeds start to turn lightly golden on the edges.
10. Remove from heat and set aside to cool.
11. In another large bowl, combine the prepared romaine, carrots, cabbage, radishes and cranberries.
12. Add them to the bowl as well when the quinoa and the sunflower is ready.
13. In a blender, combine olive oil, lime juice, rice vinegar, cilantro, maple syrup, garlic, sea salt, and chipotle chili powder.
14. Blend well, pausing to scrape down the sides.
15. Taste and adjust accordingly.

16. Drizzle in enough dressing to lightly coat the salad once tossed.

17. Serve and enjoy.

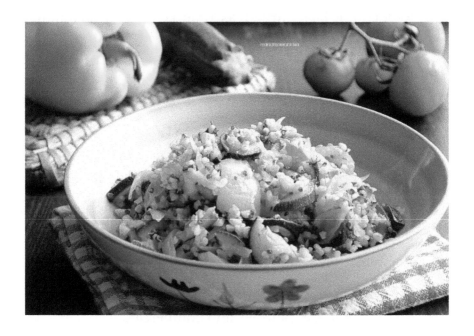

Southwestern kale power salad with sweet potato, quinoa, and avocado sauce

Ingredients

For the Quinoa and kale

- ½ teaspoon of salt
- 1 medium lime, juiced
- 1 cup of quinoa
- 2 tablespoons of olive oil
- 1 bunch of kale, ribs removed and chopped

For the Sweet potatoes

- 2 medium sweet potatoes
- 1 ½ teaspoons of salt
- 2 tablespoons of olive oil
- 1 teaspoon of smoked paprika
- 2 teaspoons of ground cumin

For the Avocado sauce

- ⅓ cup of crumbled feta, omit for vegan
- ¼ cup of pepitas
- Salt
- 2 avocados, sliced into long strips

- 2 limes, juiced
- 1 handful cilantro leaves
- ½ teaspoon of ground coriander
- 2 tablespoons olive oil
- 1 can of black beans, rinsed and drained
- 1 medium jalapeño, deseeded, membranes removed

Directions

1. Clean the quinoa and in a medium-sized pot, combine the rinsed quinoa and 2 cups water.
2. Bring the mixture to a gentle boil covered.
3. Lower the heat to a simmer let cook for 15 minutes.
4. Remove the quinoa from heat source and let rest covered for 5 minutes.
5. Uncover the pot, drain off any excess water and fluff the quinoa with a fork.
6. Set it aside to cool.
7. In another large skillet, warm the olive oil over medium heat.
8. Add the chopped sweet potatoes and toss to coat.
9. Add the cumin together with the smoked paprika and salt. Stir to combine.
10. Add a scant ¼ cup of water and cover the pan once the pan is sizzling.
11. Lower the heat to avoid burning the contents.

12. Let cook as you keep stirring occasionally, until the sweet potato is tender.

13. Raise the heat when uncovered to medium let cook until the excess moisture has evaporated in 7 minutes and the sweet potatoes are caramelizing on the edges. Let cool.

14. Transfer the kale to a large mixing bowl.

15. Sprinkle the chopped kale with salt and massage with your hands

16. Whisk together 2 tablespoons olive oil, the juice of 1 lime and ½ teaspoon salt.

17. Drizzle over the kale and toss to coat.

18. Combine the avocados, lime juice, olive oil, jalapeno, cilantro leaves, coriander, and salt in a blender.

19. Blend well then season with salt.

20. In a small skillet over medium-low heat, toast the pepitas, stirring frequently, until they are turning lightly golden on the edges in 5 minutes.

21. Once the quinoa has cooled down a bit, pour it into the bowl of kale and toss to combine.

22. Divide the kale and quinoa mixture into four large salad bowls.

23. Top with sweet potatoes, black beans, a big dollop of avocado sauce, and a sprinkle of feta and pepitas.

24. Serve and enjoy.

Sundried tomato Caesar salad

Ingredients

For the parmesan crusted croutons

- ½ cup of grated Parmesan
- 3 tablespoons of olive oil
- 2 cups of ¾-inch cubes of rustic bread
- ¼ teaspoon of salt

For the sundried tomato dressing

- Pinch sea salt
- ½ cup of grated Parmesan
- 2 tablespoons of freshly squeezed lemon juice
- Freshly ground black pepper
- ¼ cup of roughly chopped sun-dried tomatoes
- ½ cup of extra-virgin olive oil
- 2 tablespoons of water
- 1 garlic clove, roughly chopped

For the Caesar salad

- Sprinkle of additional chopped sun-dried tomatoes
- Sprinkle of additional Parmesan
- 2 small heads of romaine

Directions

1. Begin by soaking the sundried tomatoes boiling water until they're pliable, then pat them dry.
2. Next, preheat your oven to 400°F with a rack in the top of the oven.
3. Line a baking sheet with parchment paper.
4. Mix the olive oil together with the Parmesan and salt in a large mixing bowl until a paste is formed.
5. Add the cubed bread and mix well with a spatula, until all the bread is coated.
6. Turn the bread onto the prepared baking sheet and arrange in a single layer.
7. Let bake for 10 minutes, then stir and put the croutons back into the oven until they are golden brown in more 5 minutes.
8. Combine the sun-dried tomatoes together with the Parmesan, lemon juice, water, garlic and a pinch of salt in a food processor.
9. Blend briefly for 1 minute, stopping to scrape down the sides if needed.
10. While running the machine, drizzle in the olive oil and blend for 10 more seconds.
11. Taste and adjust accordingly. Set aside.
12. Drizzle the dressing over your halved romaine.
13. Finish with croutons and a sprinkle of Parmesan and sun-dried tomatoes.

14. Serve and enjoy immediately.

Chorizo tomato and charred corn salad

Ingredients

- Cayenne pepper
- 3 Spanish Chorizo sausage links, casings removed
- 1 teaspoon of sumac
- 1 loaf of rustic country
- Salt and pepper
- 2 garlic cloves, sliced
- Dried mint or parsley flakes
- 1 corn on the cob
- olive oil
- 3 tablespoon of aged white wine vinegar
- 2 large tomatoes
- 1 shallot, sliced
- 1 cup of baby spinach

Directions

1. Begin by heating a cast iron grill.
2. Add the corn to the hot skillet and grill, rotating on all sides, until it is nicely charred.
3. Remove from the skillet and let cool.

4. Place a small bowl, in a large salad bowl.

5. After the corn has cooled enough to handle, place it on top of the small bowl and, with a sharp knife, begin to slice through the kernels.

6. Set the large bowl with the corn kernels aside for later.

7. Turn the heat to medium-high.

8. Add 2 tablespoon of olive oil to the cast iron skillet.

9. In the heated oil, brown the Chorizo sausage as you toss frequently, until fully cooked.

10. Add the garlic slices and toss briefly.

11. Remove the skillet from the heat.

12. Stir in the white wine vinegar. Set aside.

13. Add the tomato wedges together with the baby spinach, shallots and spices.

14. Drizzle with olive oil toss.

15. Add the cooked Chorizo with the garlic and vinegar, toss.

16. Taste and adjust the seasoning accordingly.

17. Transfer to serving bowls and garnish with dried mint flakes.

18. Serve and enjoy with rustic bread.

Tangy lentil salad with dill and pepperoncini

Ingredients

- ½ cup of chopped pickled pepperoncini pepper
- 1 ½ cups of black beluga lentils
- ½ cup of tiny cubes of Havarti
- 2 tablespoons of tahini
- 1 bay leaf
- Freshly ground black pepper
- ¼ cup of fresh dill leaves, tough stems removed
- ⅓ cup of extra-virgin olive oil
- 2 cups of grated carrots
- ½ teaspoon of red pepper flakes
- ¼ cup of fresh dill leaves, tough stems removed
- ½ cup of chopped celery
- ½ cup of thinly sliced green onion
- ¼ cup of lemon juice
- 1 clove garlic, roughly chopped
- ¾ cup of fresh flat-leaf parsley
- Fine sea salt

Directions

1. Fill a large saucepan with water and boil over high heat.
2. When the water is boiling, add the rinsed lentils.
3. Add the bay leaf and salt.
4. Set the timer for 16 minutes.
5. Reduce the heat to prevent overflow and maintain lively simmer.
6. Combine the olive oil together with the dill, lemon juice, garlic, tahini, salt, red pepper flakes and several twists of black pepper.
7. Blend until smooth, set aside for later.
8. When the time is up, scoop out a few lentils and test for doneness.
9. Strain off all the excess water in the lentil.
10. Pour the lentils into a medium serving bowl as you discard the bay leaf.
11. Pour in all of the dressing, stir to combine.
12. Add the grated carrots together with the parsley, celery, green onion, the remaining dill, and pepperoncini peppers.
13. When the lentils are warm, add the optional cheese.
14. Stir the mixture to combine.
15. Season to taste accordingly.
16. Let it sit for 20 minutes.
17. Serve and enjoy.
18. Keep the left over refrigerated.

Mustard potato salad, Mediterranean style

The recipe contains fresh dill, parsley, red onions as well as caper for a great Mediterranean diet.

The Dijon mustard dressing is used to dress the potatoes when still hot for a perfect flavor absorption.

Ingredients

- Water
- ¼ cup of chopped red onions
- ½ teaspoon of ground sumac
- Teaspoon of salt
- ¼ teaspoon of ground coriander
- ¼ cup of fresh chopped parsley
- 2 tablespoons of capers
- ⅓ cup of extra virgin olive oil
- 2 tablespoons of white wine vinegar
- 1 ½ lb. small potatoes
- ¼ cup of chopped dill
- 2 teaspoon of Dijon mustard
- ½ teaspoon of black pepper

Directions

1. Wash slice potatoes thinly.
2. Place potatoes in a pot and add water to cover, boil.
3. Add salt.
4. Lower the let simmer for 6 minutes or so until tender.
5. Add vinaigrette ingredients to a small bowl and whisk until combined.
6. Remove from heat and drain well.
7. Place them in a large mixing bowl and immediately dress them with the Dijon mustard dressing, toss to coat.
8. Add onions, fresh herbs, and capers. Toss to combine.
9. Transfer the potatoes to a serving platter let settle for 1 hour.
10. Serve and enjoy.

Caponata recipe

The caponata recipe is largely are tasty salad made relish of eggplants and onions, celery as well as tomatoes to bring out the real taste of a Mediterranean Sea diet salad.

Ingredients

- Extra virgin olive oil
- 1 yellow onion chopped
- 1 red bell pepper cored and chopped
- ¼ cup of dry white wine
- 2 tablespoons of chopped fresh mint
- ¼ cup of red wine vinegar
- Kosher salt
- 2 small celery stalks thinly sliced
- Black pepper
- 2 tablespoons of capers
- ¼ cup of pitted green olives roughly chopped
- ¼ cup of raisins
- 1 large eggplant
- 2 teaspoons of honey more to your liking
- 1 bay leaf
- 1 cup of crushed tomatoes
- ¼ teaspoon of crushed red pepper flakes

- 2 tablespoons of chopped fresh parsley

Directions

1. Heat your oven to 400°F.
2. Season the eggplant cubes with salt 30 minutes to sweat out the bitterness.
3. Place the seasoned eggplant cubes on a sheet pan, add a drizzle of extra virgin olive oil, toss.
4. Roast the eggplant in the heated oven for 25 – 30 minutes.
5. Heat 2 tablespoons of extra virgin olive oil in a large skillet.
6. Add the onions together with the bell pepper, and celery.
7. Season with a pinch of kosher salt and black pepper.
8. Let cook for 7 minutes, tossing regularly.
9. Add the tomatoes together with the capers, olives, honey, raisins, bay leaf and crushed pepper flakes.
10. Pour in the vinegar and white wine. Stir to combine.
11. Simmer over low heat for 10 minutes.
12. Stir in the roasted eggplant and continue to cook for 3 minutes in the sauce.
13. Finish with fresh parsley and mint.
14. Serve and enjoy.

Blanched asparagus recipe with Mediterranean salsa

This asparagus recipe is fully parked with Mediterranean salsa with tomatoes, fresh herbs and shallots.

It can be served as an appetizer for a vegan dish.

Ingredients

- Zest of 1 lemon
- 1 garlic clove finely chopped
- ¼ cup of chopped fresh mint leaves
- 1 shallot finely chopped
- 12 oz. of cherry tomatoes chopped or halved
- ½ teaspoon of sumac
- 3 teaspoons of fresh lemon juice
- Greek extra virgin olive oil more for later
- ½ cup of chopped fresh parsley leaves
- 1 ½ lb. of Asparagus tough ends trimmed
- Water
- Salt and pepper

Directions

1. In a mixing bowl, add the tomatoes together with the shallots, garlic and herbs.
2. Season with salt, pepper, and sumac.
3. Add lemon juice and a drizzle of extra virgin olive oil. Mix and keep for later.
4. In a cooking pot, boil 8 cups of water, seasoned with 2 tablespoons of kosher salt.
5. Add the prepared asparagus. Boil for 4 minutes until tender.
6. Drain any excess water and immediately transfer to a bowl of ice water briefly to stop the cooking process.
7. Drain and let cool.
8. Arrange the asparagus on a serving platter.
9. Season with salt and pepper.
10. Add a drizzle of extra virgin olive oil and lemon zest.
11. Serve and enjoy topped with Mediterranean salsa.

Cantaloupe and mozzarella Caprese salad

Ingredients

- 1 tablespoon of white balsamic vinegar
- 1 8- ounce of container mozzarella balls
- 10 slices of prosciutto shredded into large pieces
- Kosher salt and freshly ground black pepper
- 1 cantaloupe halved and seeded
- ¼ cup of mint leaves thinly sliced
- ¼ cup of basil leaves thinly sliced
- 3 tablespoons of extra-virgin olive oil
- 1 ½ tablespoons of honey

Directions

1. Using a melon baller, scoop balls from the cantaloupe halves.
2. Add to a large bowl.
3. Add the mozzarella balls and the torn prosciutto.
4. Sprinkle with the basil and mint leaves.
5. In another small bowl, whisk the olive oil together with the honey and white balsamic vinegar.

6. Season with kosher salt and freshly ground black pepper.

7. Drizzle over the cantaloupe and toss.

8. Season with more salt and pepper, herbs to taste.

9. Serve and enjoy.

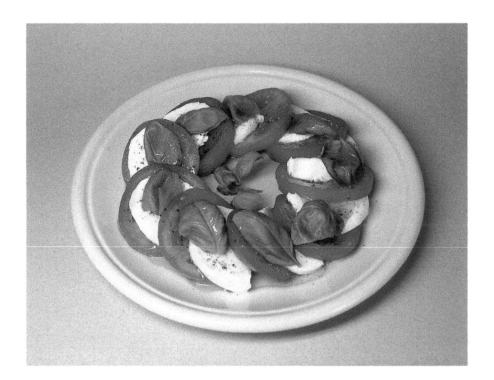

Tomato and hearts of palm salad

Ingredients

- 1 teaspoon of kosher salt
- 3 cups cherry tomatoes sliced in half
- ½ teaspoon of freshly ground black pepper
- 1 15- ounce can of hearts of palm drained and sliced.
- ¼ cup of vegetable oil
- 1 ½ tablespoon of red vinegar
- ¼ cup of thinly sliced
- 1 teaspoon of sugar
- ¼ cup of chopped Italian parsley

Directions

1. Combine tomatoes together with the hearts of palm, red onion and parsley in a large bowl.
2. In another small bowl, mix the vegetable oil with vinegar, sugar and salt and pepper until sugar is dissolved.
3. Pour vinaigrette over tomato mixture and gently mix.
4. Add more salt and pepper to taste.
5. Serve and enjoy at room temperature.

Black bean and corn salad

This black bean and corn salad features poblano pepper, fresh mind and lime giving it a unique delicious taste.

Ingredients

- ½ tsp kosher salt
- 1 cup of cherry tomatoes, halved
- 2 ears corn, cleaned with no husks
- 1 ¾ cups of cooked black beans
- 1 tablespoon of extra virgin olive oil
- ½ cup of grated coconut from frozen
- ¼ cup of lightly packed mint leaves, chopped
- 2 tablespoons of fresh lime juice
- 1 medium poblano chili

Directions

1. Wet two paper towels, squeeze out ant excess water.
2. Wrap each ear of corn in the moist paper towel and place on a dinner plate.
3. Cook in the microwave for 5 minutes.
4. Let cool briefly then carefully remove the paper towel.

5. Cut each cob in half crosswise, then stand one half at a time on a cutting board.
6. Transfer the corn kernels to a large mixing bowl.
7. Set the pablano pepper on the grates over a gas burner turned to high and use your tongs to turn the pepper until blackened in spots all over.
8. Place roasted pablano in a bowl and cover plate, let steam for 10 minutes.
9. Use your fingers to slip off the blackened skin, then remove and discard the stem and seeds.
10. Chop the roasted pablano into ½-inch pieces and add to the mixing bowl with the corn.
11. Add the black beans together with the coconut, lime juice, mint, tomatoes, olive oil and kosher salt. Toss.
12. Taste and adjust accordingly.
13. Serve and enjoy immediately.

Loaded Mediterranean chickpea salad

The manner in which the Mediterranean salad is loaded makes it a meal on its own for a Mediterranean Sea diet with a side of a perfectly roasted eggplant.

Ingredients

- Extra virgin olive oil.
- 3 tablespoons of Za'atar spice , divided
- 3 Roma tomatoes, diced
- 1 large lime, juice of
- ½ cucumber, diced
- 1 small red onion, sliced in ½ moons
- Salt and Pepper
- 1 cup cooked or canned chickpeas, drained
- 1 large eggplant, thinly sliced
- 1 cup of chopped parsley
- Salt
- 1 cup of chopped dill
- 2 garlic cloves, minced

Directions

1. Place the sliced eggplant on a large tray and sprinkle generously with salt.
2. Let it sit for 30 minutes to sweat out any bitterness.
3. Line another large tray with a paper bag topped with paper towel and place it near the stove.
4. Pat the eggplant dry.
5. Then, heat 5 tablespoons of extra virgin olive oil over medium heat until shimmering but without smoke.
6. Fry the eggplant in the oil in batches.
7. Turn over the other side when the current ones turn golden brown.
8. Remove the eggplant slices and arrange on paper towel-lined tray to drain and cool.
9. Assemble the eggplant on a serving dish.
10. Sprinkle with 1 tablespoon of Za'atar.
11. In a medium mixing bowl, combine the tomatoes, cucumbers, chickpeas, red onions, parsley and dill.
12. Add the remaining Za'atar, mix.
13. In another small bowl, whisk together the dressing.
14. Drizzle 2 tablespoons of salad dressing over the fried eggplant.
15. Pour the remaining dressing over the chickpea salad and mix.
16. Add the chickpea salad to the serving dish with the eggplant.

17. Serve and enjoy

Mediterranean chickpea faro salad with shrimp

This is an easy to make satisfying salad it entails nutty faro parked with chopped vegetables and some herbs making it largely a vegetarian diet perfect for a Mediterranean Sea diet.

Ingredients

- 1 cucumber, diced
- ½ teaspoon of sumac
- 2 green onions, trimmed and chopped
- 2 ½ cup of cooked faro
- 1 large handful fresh parsley, chopped
- 15 mint leaves, chopped
- ½ teaspoon of ground cumin
- 1 lb. large shrimp, peeled and deveined
- Kosher salt
- Black pepper
- Extra virgin olive oil
- 2 cups of cooked chickpeas, drained and rinsed
- Juice of 1 lemon
- 10 oz. of cherry tomatoes, halved
- Black pepper

- 2 teaspoons of dried oregano

Directions

1. In a small bowl, add the lemon, olive oil, salt, pepper, oregano, cumin, and sumac.
2. Whisk well.
3. In another large salad bowl, combine cooked faro together with the chickpeas and cherry tomatoes, cucumbers, green onion, parsley, and mint leaves.
4. Pour the majority of the dressing on top of the salad, toss, set aside to let the flavors melt.
5. Then, place uncooked shrimp in a bowl after patting dry with some paper towels.
6. Season with salt and pepper.
7. Drizzle extra virgin olive oil and toss to coat.
8. Heat a skillet over high heat.
9. Then, add shrimp and cook on one side till it starts to turn pink, turn over let cook 5 minutes.
10. Turn off the heat then add the remaining 3 teaspoons of dressing to the hot shrimp, toss to coat.
11. Shift to a serving platter. Make sure to add the shrimp on top.
12. Serve and enjoy.

Avocado and Greek yogurt chicken salad

Ingredients

- 1/3 cup of chopped red onion
- 1/3 cup of chopped pecans
- 1 cup of plain yogurt
- 2 tablespoons of chopped fresh tarragon
- 1 avocado, mashed
- 1-2 tablespoons fresh lemon juice
- 1/3 cup of dried cranberries
- 2 cups of shredded chicken
- ¾ cup of chopped celery
- ½ cup of red grapes, halved
- Kosher salt and freshly ground black pepper

Directions

1. In a small bowl, mix the yogurt with the avocado mash.
2. Add lemon juice.
3. Season with kosher salt and fresh ground pepper, keep aside.

4. Add the shredded chicken to the chopped celery, grapes, pecans, red onion, tarragon and cranberries to a large bowl.

5. Add the yogurt avocado sauce to the chicken mixture and toss until well combined

6. Serve and enjoy as a sandwich or appetizer.

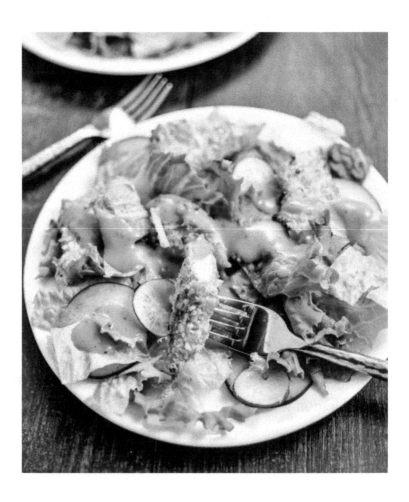

Tuscan tuna and white bean salad

Ingredients

- ¼ cup of crumbled feta cheese
- 4 cups of arugula
- 15 ounces of cannellini beans, rinsed and drained
- Kosher salt and freshly ground black pepper
- 2 tablespoons of extra virgin olive oil
- ½ cup of cherry tomatoes, halved
- ¼ cup of sliced olives
- Thinly sliced red onion
- 5 ounces of white albacore tuna packed in water
- ½ lemon

Directions

1. In a large bowl, combine the arugula together with white beans, tuna, tomatoes, olives and red onion.
2. Then, drizzle with the olive oil and the juice from the lemon. Toss.
3. Top with crumbled feta cheese.
4. Season to taste with kosher salt and black pepper.
5. Serve and enjoy.

Outrageous herbaceous Mediterranean chickpea salad

Ingredients

- 3 tablespoons of lemon juice
- 1 medium red bell pepper, chopped
- ½ teaspoon of freshly ground black pepper
- ½ teaspoon of kosher salt
- 1 ½ cups of chopped fresh flat-leaf parsley
- ½ cup of chopped red onion
- ½ cup of chopped celery plus leaves
- 3 tablespoons of extra virgin olive oil
- 2 cloves garlic, pressed
- 30 ounces of chickpeas, rinsed and drained

Directions

1. Add the chickpeas, bell pepper, parsley, red onion, and celery in a large bowl.
2. In another small bowl, whisk the olive oil with lemon juice and garlic.
3. Season to taste with the kosher salt and freshly ground black pepper.
4. Add the dressing to the chickpea mixture and toss to coat.

5. Serve and enjoy chilled.

Quinoa and burrata Caprese salad

Ingredients

- kosher salt and freshly ground black pepper
- 2 medium tomatoes sliced
- 6 basil leaves thinly sliced
- 1 packaged ball of Burrata cheese
- 2 teaspoons of balsamic vinegar
- ½ cup of quinoa cooked
- 1 ½ tablespoons of fruity extra virgin olive oil

Directions

1. Firstly, layer tomato slices in a salad bowl.
2. Remove the Burrata cheese from package and drain the water.
3. Gently tear the cheese ball in half, reserving one half for another salad.
4. Add the quinoa and basil leaves.
5. Drizzle with the olive oil and balsamic vinegar.
6. Season with the kosher salt and freshly ground pepper.
7. Serve and enjoy.

Sunshine salad dressing

Ingredients

- 2 tablespoons of lemon juice
- ½ cup of plain Greek yogurt
- ¼ cup of extra-virgin olive oil
- 2 tablespoons of apple cider vinegar
- 10 twists of freshly ground black pepper
- ½ teaspoon of fine sea salt
- ¼ cup of Dijon mustard
- 4 tablespoons of honey
- 1 clove garlic, pressed

Directions

1. In a bowl, combine all of the ingredients as listed.
2. Whisk until blended.
3. Taste and season accordingly.
4. Serve and enjoy.

Colorful chopped salad with carrots ginger dressing

Ingredients

- 6 ounces of chopped butter lettuce
- 1 ½ cups of edamame
- 1 ½ cups of chopped purple cabbage
- ¾ cup of chopped red onion
- Florets from 1 head of broccoli, finely sliced
- 1 red bell pepper, chopped
- ⅓ cup of roughly chopped fresh cilantro
- 1 batch of homemade carrot ginger dressing

Directions

1. Get a large serving bowl to combine everything apart from the dressing.
2. Toss to combine.
3. Toss in enough dressing to coat the ingredients when ready to serve.
4. Enjoy.

Pear, date and walnut salad with blue cheese

Ingredients

For the vinaigrette

- 1 ½ tablespoons white wine vinegar
- 1 teaspoon Dijon mustard
- Several twists of freshly ground black pepper
- ¼ cup extra-virgin olive oil
- Pinch of salt
- 1 teaspoon honey or maple syrup

For the salad

- ⅓ cup of crumbled blue cheese
- 7 Medjool dates, pitted and sliced thin
- ⅓ cup of chopped raw walnuts
- 6 ounces of red leaf lettuce, torn into small pieces
- 2 Bosc

Directions

Make the dressing:

1. In a small bowl, combine all of the dressing ingredients and whisk.
2. Taste, and adjust accordingly.

Make the salad:

3. Toast the walnuts in a medium skillet over medium heat until fragrant in 5 minutes, keep aside.
4. Then, in a medium serving bowl, combine the greens together with the dates, pears and toasted walnuts.
5. Drizzle with dressing and toss until the greens are lightly coated.
6. Serve and enjoy.

Crispy apple and kohlrabi salad

Ingredients

- 2 tablespoons of lemon juice, to taste
- 1 large of Honey crisp apple
- 3 tablespoons of toasted sunflower seeds
- Flaky sea salt and black pepper
- ⅓ cup of grated gouda cheese
- ¼ cup of fresh tarragon leaves
- 2 small kohlrabi
- Lemon zest
- 2 tablespoons of olive oil

Directions

1. In a large serving bowl, combine the kohlrabi and apple matchsticks.
2. Add the cheese and the tarragon leaves with sunflower seeds.
3. Shave lemon zest liberally over the bowl.
4. Drizzle in 1 tablespoon of olive oil and 1 tablespoon lemon juice.
5. Sprinkle lightly with salt and black pepper.
6. Toss with your hands.
7. Serve and enjoy.

Spicy harissa white bean and lentil salad

The spicy harissa white bean lentil salad derives its tempting taste flavor and taste from garlic and other Middle Eastern spices making a perfect Mediterranean diet.

Ingredients

- Olive oil
- 3 tablespoon of distilled white vinegar, divided
- 3 garlic cloves, chopped
- Silvered almonds toasted
- 1 14-oz. can of white beans, rinsed and drained
- 3 cups of water
- 2 ½ medium sweet onions, thinly sliced
- 4 medium tomatoes diced
- ½ teaspoon of ground coriander
- Fresh mint for garnish
- ½ teaspoon of allspice
- 1 cup of dry brown lentils, rinsed
- ½ teaspoon of sugar
- Pinch salt
- ⅓ cup of harissa paste

- 2 grated carrots

Directions

1. In a medium sauce pan, combine the lentils and water.
2. Bring to a quick simmer on medium-high heat, then lower the heat and let simmer further for 20 minutes.
3. Drain any excess water.
4. In a large cast iron skillet, heat 2 tablespoon of olive oil.
5. Add the majority of the onions.
6. Add the garlic. Toss until golden.
7. Add the tomatoes together with the spices, sugar, salt and 2 tablespoon of vinegar.
8. Let cook for 5 minutes on medium-high heat to soften the tomatoes.
9. Stir in the harissa paste and only ½ cup water.
10. Let it continue for 4 minutes, then add the boiled lentils and the white beans.
11. Stir to combine. Continue to cook for 5 more minutes.
12. Turn the heat off and stir in 1 tablespoon of distilled white vinegar.
13. Transfer the lentil salad to a serving platter. Allow it to cool shortly.
14. Cover and refrigerate until you are ready to serve.
15. Before serving, top the lentil salad with a drizzle of olive oil.

16. Add the grated carrots, ½ cup chopped onions, fresh mint and almonds.
17. Serve and enjoy with pita bread.

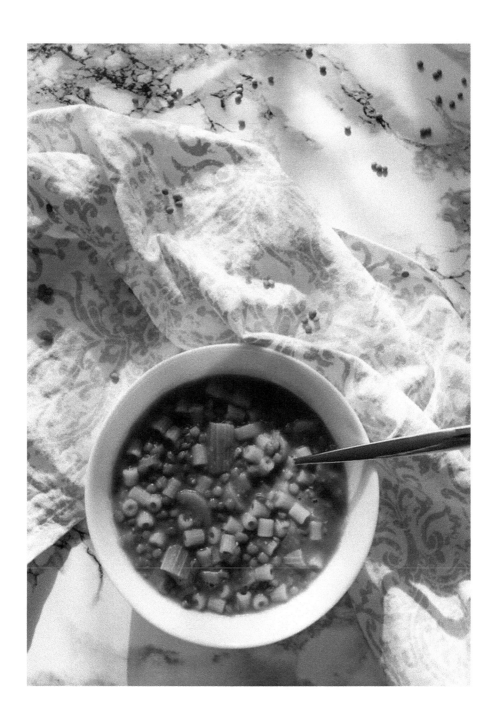